Lavender

Fragrant Herbs for Home & Bath

Gloria Hander Lyons

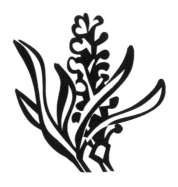

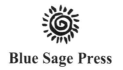

Blue Sage Press

Lavender Sensations
Fragrant Herbs for Home & Bath

Inquires should be addressed to:
Blue Sage Press
48 Borondo Pines
La Marque, TX 77568
www.BlueSagePress.com

ISBN: 978-0-9790618-8-2

Library of Congress Control Number: 2007908075

First Edition: November, 2007

Printed in the United States of America

Table of Contents

Lavender has been a favorite herb for centuries. During ancient times, the Greeks and Romans bathed in lavender-scented water. The name lavender comes from the Latin word "lavare" which means "to wash".

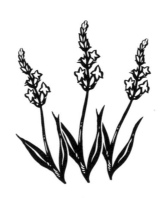

Lavender Sensations: Fragrant Herbs for Home & Bath

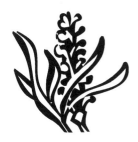

A field of lavender is a beautiful sight to behold. Its fragrant, purple flowers, soothing aroma and distinctive flavor make it desirable for crafting hundreds of products for personal, culinary or household use.

You can use it to concoct a relaxing herbal bath mixture, a stimulating beauty scrub, or a soothing foot soak.

Its aroma can help reduce stress, encourage sleep or relieve headaches when used in the form of herbal sleep pillows or eye pillows.

Sachets, a smaller version of sleep pillows, can scent your linens, perfume your lingerie drawer or repel bugs in your closets.

Lavender potpourris or pomanders introduce a wonderful fragrance to your home or closets.

You can also use lavender for crafting a wide range of culinary dishes. French chefs have used it for centuries to add its sweet, floral flavor to their cuisine.

Spark your gift-giving creativity and delight your friends, family and co-workers when you present them with delicious lavender-flavored treats and mixes.

This book includes more than 40 craft projects and recipes for using dried lavender to make bath and body products that help promote relaxation, plus fragrant sachets and potpourri's to scent your home, and delectable goodies for gifts.

If you're an avid gardener, growing and drying your own lavender is easy to do. Not only will you reap the benefits of this beautiful, fragrant herb for personal, culinary and household use, it will add beauty outside your home, as well.

Growing your own lavender is not a requirement, however; you can buy dried lavender buds for use in cooking and crafting. Just make sure the herbs you purchase have not been sprayed with any pesticides.

If you don't have a local source for buying dried lavender and other herbs for making the projects in this book, you can find mail order sources through the Internet. A couple of sources that I have used are listed in the ordering information following the index.

Whether you're crafting soothing bath and body products or mixing up a tasty recipe, lavender is a welcome and versatile herb to have on hand.

Lavender Bath
& Body Products

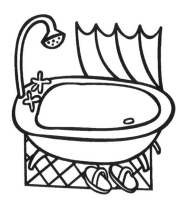

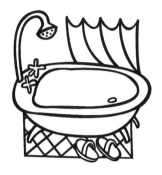

Lavender Bath & Body Products

Everyone enjoys a relaxing, hot bath, but adding fragrant herbs to the steamy water makes bathing a luxurious treat.

You can customize the bath to your needs, whether it's relaxing, stimulating, soothing, moisturizing or simply fragrant, by changing the herbs in your bath mixture:

- For a relaxing bath, use a blend of the following herbs: lavender, chamomile, lemon verbena or roses.

- For an energizing bath, stir up a mixture of these herbs: lavender, rosemary, peppermint, rose geranium, jasmine or lemon balm.

- For an all-purpose herbal bath, combine equal amounts of lavender, rosemary, peppermint, lemon verbena and roses.

Bath Time Tip: Never add loose herbs directly to the bath water. They will stick to your skin, as well as the sides of the tub, and may also clog your drain.

There are three methods for preparing herbal baths:

- Infusion: Pour 4 cups of boiling water over 1/4 cup of herbs and steep for 15-20 minutes. Strain the herb-infused water and add it to your bath water.

- Decoction: Boil 1/4 cup of herbs in 1 cup of water for 20 minutes. Strain and add to the bath water.

- Bath Bag: Place several tablespoons of herbs in a small muslin drawstring bag and hang the bag from the tub faucet under the running water. You can also add the bag to the water and rub it on your skin while bathing.

NOTE: Allergic reactions can occur with any herbal ingredient. Be sure to test any bath mixture on a small area of skin before using in the bath. Pregnant women should avoid using homemade herbal products. Make sure the herbs you use have not been sprayed with any pesticides.

Try crafting a few of the following bath and body products for your own personal use or to give as gifts to family or friends.

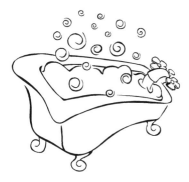

Soothing Lavender Oatmeal Bath

Adding oatmeal to this bath mixture helps to moisturize the skin.

1 cup oatmeal
1/2 cup cornmeal
1/2 cup dried lavender buds
1/4 cup dried rosemary
2 tablespoons powdered milk

Process oatmeal in a food processor until finely ground. Add remaining ingredients and process until well blended. Store in an airtight container.

To Use: Fill a small draw-string muslin bag with about 2 tablespoons of the mixture. Place under faucet while running the water for your bath.

You can also toss the bag into the bath water and rub it on your skin while bathing.

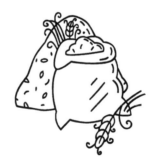

Romantic Lavender & Rose Bath

This bath blend makes a wonderful gift when presented in an attractive glass canister. Not only is it relaxing, but it leaves your skin scented with just a hint of lavender and roses.

1 cup oatmeal
1/2 cup dried lavender buds
1/2 cup dried rose petals
1/4 cup dried chamomile

Process the oatmeal in a food processor until finely ground.

Add remaining ingredients and process until well blended. Store in an airtight container.

To Use: Fill a small draw-string muslin bag with about 2 tablespoons of the mixture. Place under faucet while running the water for your bath.

You can also toss the bag into the bath water and rub it on your skin while bathing.

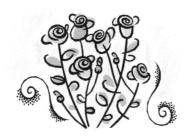

Lavender Bath Salts

1/2 cup dried lavender buds
1/4 cup dried lemon verbena
1/2 cup baking soda
1/2 cup Epsom salt

Blend all ingredients together and place in an airtight container.

To Use: Fill a small draw-string muslin bag with about 2 or 3 tablespoons of the mixture.

Place under the faucet while running the water for your bath. Then toss the bag into the bath water while bathing.

To give as a gift, place mixture in an attractive canister or tin. Attach the instructions for using the bath salts. Include a small wooden scoop and a few muslin drawstring bags with your gift.

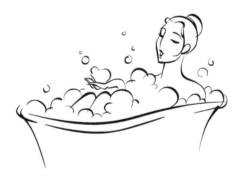

Lavender Soap

Lavender flowers are antiseptic and relaxing and therefore, the perfect choice for soap. The fragrance of lavender is a classic scent that will never go out of style.

This soap is simple and quick to make, using white, opaque melt and pour soap found at your local craft store.

4 oz. (about 4 squares) of white, opaque melt and pour soap
1 teaspoon ground, dried lavender buds
3 drops red soap dye (do not use food coloring)
1 drop blue soap dye
2 drops lavender fragrance oil for soap (optional)
1 (2-1/2" X 3-1/2") oval or rectangular soap mold

Lightly coat the inside of your soap mold with cooking oil. Cut soap into 1/2" cubes and place in a 1 cup glass measuring cup. Microwave on high power 30-40 seconds until melted.

Using a wooden spoon or craft stick, stir in lavender. Add dye and fragrance oil if desired. Stir slowly to avoid creating bubbles in your soap mixture.

Pour soap mixture into soap mold. Let cool 30-40 minutes before removing from mold. Use your thumbs to apply gentle pressure to release the soap from the mold. If difficult to remove, place in the refrigerator or freezer for 10 minutes.

Wrap soap in plastic wrap immediately after removing from mold. Storing your soap in plastic until ready to use will help retain its fragrance. Cure soap at least 48 hours before using.

Lavender Oatmeal Soap

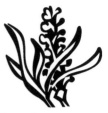

Adding oatmeal to your soap helps make it more moisturizing and adds the benefit of exfoliating properties.

4 oz. (about 4 squares) of white, opaque melt and pour soap
1-1/2 teaspoons oatmeal, finely ground in a food processor
1 teaspoon ground, dried lavender buds
3 drops red soap dye (do not use food coloring)
1 drop blue soap dye
2 drops lavender fragrance oil for soap (optional)
1 (2-1/2" X 3-1/2") oval or rectangular soap mold

Lightly coat the inside of your soap mold with cooking oil. Cut soap into 1/2" cubes and place in a 1 cup glass measuring cup. Microwave on high power 30-40 seconds until melted.

Using a wooden spoon or craft stick, stir in lavender and oatmeal. Add dye and fragrance oil if desired. Stir slowly to avoid creating bubbles in your soap mixture.

NOTE: To prevent the oatmeal from sinking to the bottom of the mold, cool soap mixture slightly, stirring occasionally, before pouring into mold.

Pour soap mixture into soap mold. Let cool 30-40 minutes before removing from mold. Use your thumbs to apply gentle pressure to release the soap from the mold. If difficult to remove, place in the refrigerator or freezer for 10 minutes.

Wrap soap in plastic wrap immediately after removing from mold. Storing your soap in plastic until ready to use will help retain its fragrance. Cure soap at least 48 hours before using.

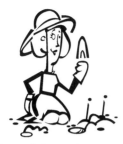

Lavender Gardener's Soap

Adding cornmeal and dried lemon peel to this soap makes it just abrasive enough for removing dirt from your hands after gardening.

4 oz. (about 4 squares) of white, opaque melt and pour soap
1 teaspoon cornmeal
1/2 teaspoon ground, dried lavender buds
1/2 teaspoon ground, dried chamomile flowers
1/2 teaspoon dried, grated lemon peel
3 drops red soap dye (do not use food coloring)
1 drop blue soap dye
1 (2-1/2" X 3-1/2") oval or rectangular soap mold

Lightly coat the inside of soap mold with cooking oil. Cut soap into 1/2" cubes and place in a 1 cup glass measuring cup. Microwave on high power 30-40 seconds until melted. Using a wooden spoon or craft stick, stir in lavender, chamomile, lemon peel and cornmeal. Add dye and fragrance oil if desired. Stir slowly to avoid creating bubbles in soap mixture. NOTE: To prevent the cornmeal from sinking to the bottom of the mold, cool soap mixture slightly, stirring occasionally, before pouring into mold.

Pour soap mixture into soap mold. Let cool 30-40 minutes before removing from mold. Use your thumbs to apply gentle pressure to release the soap from the mold. If difficult to remove, place in the refrigerator or freezer for 10 minutes.

Wrap soap in plastic wrap immediately after removing from mold. Storing your soap in plastic until ready to use will help retain its fragrance. Cure soap at least 48 hours before using.

Lavender Shower Bags

These little bags can be used in the shower in case you don't have time to soak in the bath tub.

1/4 cup oatmeal
3 tablespoons dried lavender buds
1 tablespoon dried rosemary
2 tablespoons grated soap (Ivory or Dove)

Combine all ingredients in a small bowl and stir until well blended. Store mixture in an airtight container.

To use: Place about 2 tablespoons of the mixture in a terrycloth drawstring bag, or bundle 2 tablespoons of the mixture into a washcloth and secure with string. Use the bag in the shower to wash your body.

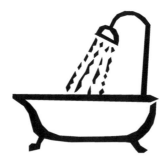

Lavender Tea Bags for the Bath

Green tea is not only a healthy drink, it adds a refreshing scent to the bath. It is especially soothing when combined with the relaxing qualities of lavender and skin softening properties of chamomile.

1/2 cup loose green tea
1/4 cup dried lavender buds
1/4 cup dried chamomile flowers

Blend all ingredients together and store in an airtight container.

To Use: Fill a small draw-string muslin bag with about 3 tablespoons of the mixture. In a small sauce pan, bring 2 cups of water to a boil. Place the tea bag in the pan of water, cover, remove from heat and let steep for 15-20 minutes. Then add the tea and tea bag to your bath water and enjoy.

To give as a gift: Place several bath tea bags in an attractive tin or in a plastic zipper-type bag that is tucked inside a fabric gift bag (see page 51 for instructions for making fabric bags). Attach instructions for using.

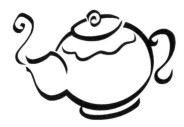

Lavender Beauty Scrub

Facial scrubs made of grated soap and dried herbs cleanse, stimulate and soothe the skin. They are simple to make and attractive when displayed in a glass container.

1/2 cup grated soap (Dove or Ivory)
1/2 cup oatmeal
1/2 cup dried lavender buds
1/2 cup dried sage leaves
1/4 cup dried mint leaves

Blend all ingredients together. Store mixture in an airtight container.

To use: Place 2 to 3 tablespoons of the mixture into a small muslin draw-string bag or bundle into a washcloth. Wet the bag and rub over your face or body with a gentle circular motion.

Lavender Sugar Body Scrub

This recipe is intended to be mixed right before using.

1/4 cup granulated sugar
1 tablespoon ground, dried lavender buds
2 tablespoons vegetable oil
2 tablespoons whole milk

Blend the ingredients together into a smooth cream.

To use: Massage mixture all over the body to increase circulation and remove dry, flaky skin.

Rinse with warm water. Dry off and then apply a good skin moisturizer.

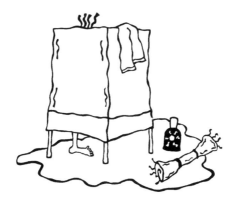

Lavender Foot Soak

This mixture is a luxurious treat for tired feet. It makes an extra special gift for someone who must stand throughout most of their workday. Present it in an attractive canister or place the mixture in a plastic zipper-type bag and tuck inside a fabric gift bag (see instructions for making gift bags on page 51). Attach instructions for using and include a small wooden scoop and several muslin drawstring bags.

1/4 cup dried lavender buds
2 tablespoons dried rosemary
2 tablespoons dried sage
2 tablespoons Epsom salt

In a small bowl, combine all ingredients and stir until well blended. Store in an airtight container or plastic zipper-type bag.

To use: Place 2-3 tablespoons of the mixture in a small drawstring bag. Steep in very warm water in a foot-soaking tub for 5 minutes before soaking your feet. Leave the bag in the water while soaking.

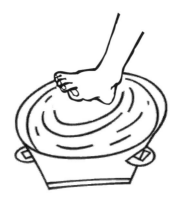

Lavender
Aroma Therapy

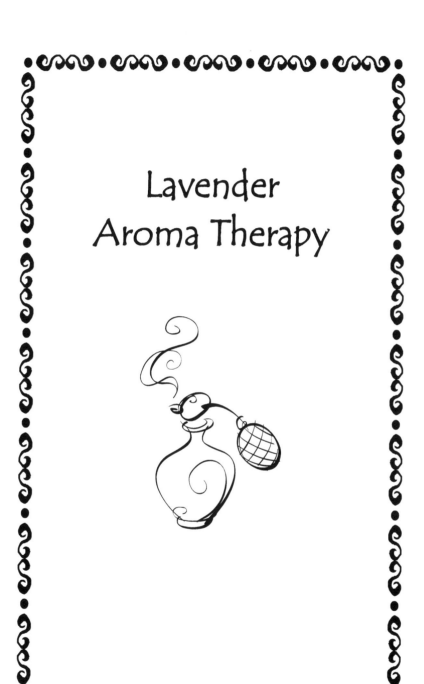

Lavender
Aroma Therapy

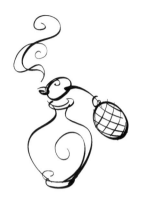

Lavender is grown commercially for the production of lavender essential oil. Its fragrance is one of the most important aromas in aromatherapy because of its "balancing" properties. It can be energizing or calming, revitalizing or relaxing.

Fresh or dried, lavender has many uses in the home. A bouquet of lavender is not only a beautiful decoration, it adds a wonderful fragrance to your room.

Alone or combined with other herbs, dried lavender can be used to make scented pillows to encourage restful sleep. You can use lavender sachets to perfume linen closets and lingerie drawers.

Other herbs blended with lavender in the form of potpourris can add a pleasant fragrance to the air or ward off unwanted pests in your closets or carpets.

Try a few of the following craft projects to experience of the soothing scent of lavender.

Lavender Sleep Pillow

For a fragrant pillow to promote restful sleep, use dried lavender or a mixture of dried herbs and flowers such as chamomile, lavender, marjoram and rose petals.

To make the pillow, sew two 8" squares of muslin together, right sides facing each other, along three sides, using a 1/4" seam allowance.

Turn the pillow right side out and fill with about 3/4 cup of lavender or the herb mixture of your choice, to make a very thin pillow. Turn under the raw edges of the open side 1/4" and stitch closed.

To use, tuck the sleep pillow inside the pillow case on your bed pillow and enjoy the relaxing fragrance of lavender.

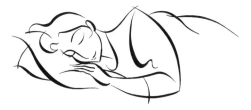

Headache Pillows

Headache pillows were popular in Victorian times. These small pillows, filled with lavender and placed under the back of the neck while reclining were commonly used to relieve headaches.

You can try one for yourself. Follow the directions for making the sleep pillow on page 19, using two pieces of fabric about 4-1/2" X 8-1/2" to make a rectangular-shaped pillow to fit the back of your neck. Choose a luxurious fabric like satin or velvet.

Make a separate herb pouch from two 3-1/2" squares of muslin fabric, following the directions for the sleep pillow. Fill with about 1/4 cup of dried lavender turn under the raw edges on the open end and stitch the opening closed.

Stuff your pillow using polyester batting and tuck the herb pouch inside. Turn under the raw edges of your pillow 1/4" and sew the opening closed.

Use whenever you feel the need to relax and de-stress. These pillows make thoughtful gifts for friends.

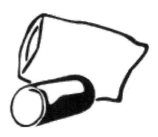

Lavender & Mint Travel Pillow

To ease stress and possible motion sickness while traveling, make a muslin pouch of the following herb mixture to insert inside the pillow case of a small travel-size pillow to use for napping or resting.

1/4 cup dried lavender buds
1/4 cup dried peppermint leaves
1/4 cup lemon verbena leaves
1 tablespoon dried, crushed lemon peel

Blend all ingredients together. To make the muslin pouch, sew two 8" squares of muslin together, right sides facing each other, along three sides, using a 1/4" seam allowance.

Turn the pouch right sides out and fill with the herb mixture. Turn under the raw edges of the open side 1/4" and stitch closed.

Tuck the pouch inside the pillow case on your travel-size pillow and enjoy the soothing aroma.

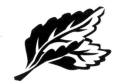

Stress Relief Eye Pillow

A stress relief eye pillow is simple to make and will relax you or help you sleep. It is a small rectangular pillow made from cotton or muslin fabric and sized to fit over both eyes.

To make an eye pillow, cut two rectangles approximately 4-1/2" X 9-1/2" from fabric. Sew the two pieces together around two long sides and one short side, with the right sides of the fabric facing each other and using a 1/4" seam allowance. Turn right sides out. Fill the pillow case loosely with a mixture of 3/4 cup dried lavender buds and 3/4 cup flax seed. Turn under the raw edges of the open end 1/4" and sew the opening closed.

If you like, you can also make a removable, washable pillow case for your eye pillow. Simply cut two fabric pieces about one inch wider and two inches longer than your eye pillow. Sew together, right sides facing each other, using a 1/4" seam allowance, leaving one end open. Turn pillow case right side out. Turn under and hem the edges of the open end of your pillow case. Slip eye pillow inside the case.

To use, lay the pillow across your eyes to relieve stress headaches, or warm it in the microwave and wrap it around your neck to reduce tension. If you chill it in the freezer, it can be used to reduce puffiness around the eyes.

These make thoughtful gifts for friends, especially when sewn from elegant satin or velvet fabrics.

Helpful Hint: To help your eye pillow retain its fragrance longer, store in a zipper-type plastic bag when not in use. Squeeze gently to release more lavender fragrance.

Sachets

Sachets are small pillows, about 2" or 3" square that are filled with aromatic herbs and used to perfume linen closets and clothes drawers. They are usually made from decorative fabrics and trimmed with ribbons and lace.

You can fill them with a mixture of herbs such as lavender and rose petals or just lavender. For a stronger scent, mix a few drops of lavender fragrance oil with the herbs before filling the sachet pillows. Sachets are easy to make and fun to give as gifts or party favors.

Helpful Hint: When your sachets start to lose their scent, squeeze them to release more of the natural oils in the herbs.

Easy Handkerchief Sachets

Pretty embroidered or lace-edged handkerchiefs make attractive sachets for your lingerie drawers. Make several to give as gifts.

Place about 1 tablespoon of dried lavender buds in the center of a handkerchief. Gather the corners together and tie a narrow satin ribbon just above the bundle of lavender to secure.

For a stronger scent and a larger sachet, add several drops of lavender fragrance oil to a cotton ball and place it in the center of the handkerchief with the dried lavender buds. Draw up the corners of the handkerchief and secure with a narrow satin ribbon.

Simple Drawstring Bag Sachets

You can purchase 3" X 4" organza drawstring bags at craft stores (usually found in the wedding and party section) for making simple, but attractive sachets to give as party favors or gifts.

Fill each bag with about 1-1/2 to 2 tablespoons of dried lavender buds or a blend of lavender and dried roses or the herbs of your choice, and tie the bag closed using the drawstrings.

If you like, use a hot glue gun to attach a small artificial flower over the drawstring ribbon knot for more decoration.

These pretty and fragrant bags make great party favors at bridal showers, anniversary celebrations or tea parties. The organza bags come in a wide variety of colors to match your party theme.

Purchase lavender-colored bags and fill with dried lavender for guest favors at a "Lavender and Lace" tea party.

Use ivory-colored bags and fill with a mixture of lavender and roses for guest favors at a bridal shower.

You can also use these bags as guest favors at weddings so the guests can toss the herbs over the bride and groom as they leave the reception. Match the bag sachets to the wedding colors and/or theme.

See page 25 for instructions for making Wedding Potpourri to fill these tiny organza bags.

Wedding Potpourri

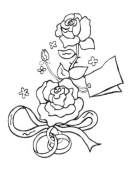

In the early 1700's, "floriography" (the language of flowers) was introduced in England, which started the popular Victorian trend of sending messages by flowers and herbs.

You can use floriography to make wedding potpourri. Simply mix the herbs or flowers that express your wishes for the bridal couple and their future together. Give each guest a small bag of the potpourri to toss over the bride and groom as they leave the celebration.

To make the potpourri, blend together the following ingredients:

1 cup dried lavender buds (devotion)
1-1/2 cups dried rose petals (love)
1 cup dried chamomile flowers (patience)
1/2 cup dried rosemary leaves (remembrance)
1/2 cup dried marjoram leaves (joy)
1/2 cup dried sage leaves (wisdom)

Fill 3" X 4" organza drawstring bags with a rounded tablespoon of the mixture. Or place a rounded tablespoon of the potpourri into the center of a 9" tulle circle and tie closed with satin ribbon. Recipe makes about 50 guest bags.

Arrange the bags in a pretty basket with a sign that says: This wedding potpourri contains lavender for devotion, rosemary for remembrance, marjoram for joy, sage for wisdom, roses for love and chamomile for patience.

A few more floriography meanings are listed below:

Allspice	Compassion
Basil	Good Wishes
Caraway	Faithfulness
Chervil	Sincerity
Cloves	Dignity
Daisy	Innocence
Lemon Balm	Sympathy
Thyme	Happiness
Violet	Faith

This potpourri can also be used for an anniversary celebration. Create a special blend of herbs, flowers and spices for the couple you are honoring, to express your wishes for their future together. Place the potpourri into 3" X 4" organza bags to give as favors to your guests.

Follow the instructions for the wedding potpourri and place the favors in a decorative basket with a sign to let guests know the significance of the fragrant blend.

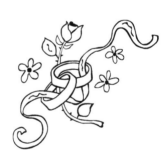

Lavender
Household
Products

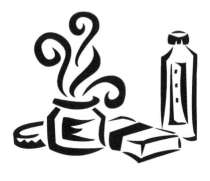

Lavender Clothes Dryer Sachets

Freshen your sheets and clothes with the lovely scent of lavender. Make simple dryer sachets to toss into the dryer while drying your laundry.

To make each sachet: Cut two, 4" squares of cotton muslin. Stack the two fabric pieces, right sides facing each other, and sew around three sides, using a 1/4" seam allowance. Turn the bag right side out. Fill with 1/3 cup dried lavender buds, turn under the edges of the open end 1/4" and stitch the opening closed. Store in an airtight container to help retain their fragrance.

To use, toss in the dryer for the last 15 minutes of the cycle to add the fresh scent of lavender to your linens and clothes.

These sachets can be reused 3 or 4 times. Squeeze them gently before each use to release more of the natural oils.

After using them in the dryer, store them with your linens, blankets or clothes. Not only will they scent your stored items, but lavender is a natural moth repellant.

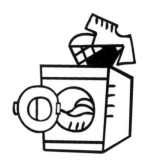

Lavender Sachets for Your Car

Does your car smell like stale junk food, or worse, last week's work-out clothes from the gym? Replace those unpleasant odors with the fresh scent of lavender.

The relaxing aroma of lavender can also help relieve stress during those long rush-hour traffic commutes.

To make each sachet: Cut two, 4" squares of cotton muslin fabric. Stack the two fabric pieces, right sides facing each other, and sew around three sides, using a 1/4" seam allowance. Turn the bag right side out. Fill with 1/3 cup of dried lavender buds, turn under the edges of the open end 1/4" and stitch the opening closed.

Stash a couple of these sachets underneath your car seats for a refreshing change.

When the sachets start to loose their scent, squeeze them gently to release more of the natural oils in the herbs.

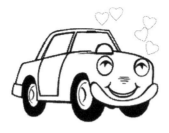

Bug Repelling Closet Sachet

These sachets will help repel moths, fleas, silverfish, and other unwanted pests in your closets, while adding a fresh, fragrant scent. To make the potpourri to fill one sachet, you will need:

3 tablespoons cedar wood chips
3 tablespoons dried lavender buds
1 teaspoon coarsely chopped cinnamon sticks
1/4 teaspoon whole cloves
1/4 teaspoon whole black peppercorns

Blend all ingredients together.

To make each sachet: Cut two, 4" squares of cotton print fabric. Stack the two fabric pieces, right sides facing each other, and sew around three sides, using a 1/4" seam allowance. Turn the bag right side out. Fill with the potpourri, turn under the raw edges of the open end of the bag 1/4" and stitch the opening closed.

Using a 6" length of 1/2" wide satin or grosgrain ribbon, attach a hanger to one side of the bag (see the picture on the front cover). Hang the sachet from a clothes hanger in your closet

Lavender & Herb Hot Pad

Rest a warm teapot or bowl of soup on this pad to release its spicy fragrance. (Do not place extremely hot pans on this pad—they can scorch the fabric.)

2 (6") squares of cotton muslin fabric
2 (8") squares of homespun or cotton print fabric
2 (8") squares of thin polyester quilt batting

Spice mixture to fill muslin bag: 1/4 cup dried lavender buds, 3 tablespoons dried sage leaves, 2 tablespoons dried marjoram leaves, 1 tablespoon coarsely crushed cinnamon sticks, 1 tablespoon dried orange peel and 1 teaspoon whole cloves. (Or use any combination of herbs and spices of your choice to equal about 3/4 cup.)

Muslin Spice Bag: Using a 1/4" seam allowance, sew the two muslin squares together around three sides of the square, right-sides facing each other. Turn the bag right side out. Fill with the herb and spice mixture. Turn under the raw edges of the open side of the bag 1/4" and stitch the opening closed.

Hot Pad: Stack the two batting squares on top of each other. Lay one homespun fabric square on top of the batting squares, right side up. Lay the remaining homespun square on top of the stack, right side down. Pin all layers together. Using a 3/8" seam allowance, sew the stack of squares together around three sides. Turn the bag right side out with both layers of batting inside the homespun fabric bag.

Slip the muslin bag filled with herbs and spices inside the homespun bag, between the two layers of batting. Turn under the raw edges of the open side of the hot pad 3/8" and stitch the opening closed.

Lavender & Herb Mug Mat

Keep this mug mat on your desk to rest your warm coffee or tea mug. The energizing scent from this herbal blend will help keep you alert. Make several to give to friends and co-workers.

2 (5") squares of cotton print or homespun fabric
3 tablespoons dried lavender buds
2 tablespoons dried peppermint leaves
2 tablespoons dried sage leaves
2 teaspoons dried, grated lemon peel
2 tablespoons flaxseed for filler

Using a 1/4" seam allowance, sew the two cotton squares together, right sides facing each other, around three sides of the square. Turn the bag right side out.

In a small bowl, blend the herbs and filler together. Pour the mixture into the cotton bag. Turn under the raw edges of the open end of the bag 1/4" and stitch the opening closed.

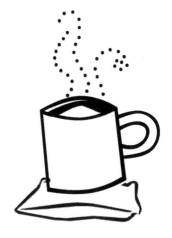

Lavender Pomander

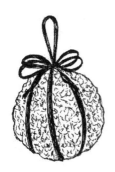

Cover Styrofoam spheres with dried lavender buds and decorate with ribbons to make a fragrant pomander.

Hang them up to scent your closets or give them as gifts.

To make a lavender pomander you will need the following:

Dried lavender buds
White craft glue
3" Styrofoam balls
Ribbons & straight pins

Spread the lavender buds out onto wax paper. Coat one half of a Styrofoam ball with a thick layer of white craft glue. Roll it in lavender buds. Let dry. Repeat on the opposite half of the ball and place on wax paper to dry. Decorate the pomander with ribbons and add a ribbon hanging loop secured by straight pins.

Lavender & Rose Pomander

For a slightly sweeter smelling pomander, follow the instructions above using a mixture of half dried lavender buds and half dried, crushed rose petals.

Spicy Lavender Pomanders

You can make a spicy version of the lavender pomander to add a fragrant scent to your kitchen. These pomanders are not hung, but placed in a small, attractive bowl or serving dish on your kitchen counter. They will scent the entire room.

1/4 cup dried lavender buds
1 tablespoon whole cloves
2 tablespoons cinnamon sticks, finely crushed
2 teaspoons dried orange peel, crushed
3 (2-1/2") Styrofoam balls
White craft glue

Mix the herbs and spices together in a bowl. Coat one half of a Styrofoam ball with a thick layer of white craft glue. Sprinkle the herb mixture over the glue and press in place. Place on wax paper to dry. Repeat on the opposite half of the ball and let dry.

Lavender Christmas Ornaments

These ornaments will not only decorate your tree, but scent the room as well. Purchase clear glass Christmas ball ornaments. Remove the hanger and fill the glass ball ornaments about half full with dried lavender. Reattach the hanger. Slip a length of 1" wide purple organza ribbon through the hanging wire and tie a bow. These ornaments make nice Christmas gifts.

They also make great party favors. Write your guests' names on the glass balls using a gold metallic paint pen and they can do double duty as place cards when nestled into a pretty candle wreath and placed beside each guest's place setting.

Lavender Carpet Freshener

1-1/2 cups dried lavender buds
1 cup dried rosemary leaves
1 cup baking soda

Mix all the ingredients together until well blended. Store the mixture in an airtight container.

To use: Sprinkle carpet freshener blend lightly over carpet. Leave for a about an hour, then vacuum.

This herbal blend adds a nice fragrance that can deodorize your carpet and helps to repel moths, fleas and pet odors.

The herbs in the vacuum cleaner bag will also scent your room while you vacuum them up.

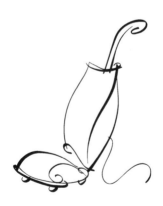

Lavender & Herb Fire Starter Bundles

What could be cozier than a blazing fire in the fireplace on a cold winter evening? How about adding the pleasing, natural scent of herbs?

After stripping the leaves and flowers off fragrant herbs and flowers, like lavender, sage, rosemary, mint and eucalyptus, save the leftover stems to use in fire starter bundles.

Simply gather together a hand full of stems, about 1-1/2" in diameter. Tie them together using natural raffia and let them dry.

Toss one on the fire in your fireplace and enjoy the fragrant scent.

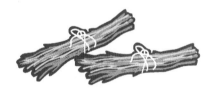

Culinary
Crafting
with Lavender

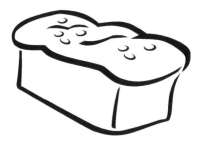

Culinary Crafting with Lavender

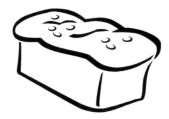

Not only is lavender an excellent choice for making relaxing bath and body mixtures and fragrant household products, it can add a deliciously distinctive flavor to your cooking.

Lavender is a member of the mint family. It tastes very similar to rosemary, with a sweet, floral flavor and just a hint of citrus.

The secret to cooking with lavender is: a little goes a long way. It has a strong flavor, so use it sparingly. Adding too much lavender to your recipe will make it bitter.

Try crafting a few of the following recipes to give as gifts or for your own enjoyment.

IMPORTANT NOTE: Make sure that the lavender you use for cooking has not been sprayed with any pesticides. It should be labeled **"FOR CULINARY USE"**.

Contraindications and Safety: It is recommended that lavender be avoided if you are pregnant or nursing. Also, it should not to be used with preparations containing iron and/or iodine. If you are taking prescription medications, check with your physician about possible contraindications for any herb.

Lavender & Lace Tea

Packets of Lavender & Lace Tea make nice favors for tea parties when bundled in a pretty lace handkerchief and tied with satin ribbon. Be sure to attach the instructions for preparing the tea.

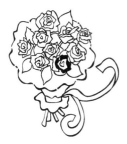

1/2 teaspoon dried lavender buds (labeled for culinary use)
1 teaspoon dried rose petals (labeled for culinary use)
2 tablespoons black tea leaves

Blend ingredients together and store in an airtight container. If giving as a gift, place in a plastic zipper-type bag and tuck inside a pretty handkerchief as described above or use an 8" square of pretty fabric.

This recipe makes one six-cup pot of tea. Place tea mixture into a warmed teapot. Add six cups of boiling water and steep for 3 to 5 minutes. Strain into cups.

Sweeten with honey or sugar if desired.

Lavender & Vanilla Hot Cocoa Mix

1/2 cup instant nonfat dry milk
3 tablespoons granulated sugar
2 tablespoons unsweetened cocoa powder
1-1/2 tablespoons powdered French Vanilla flavored
    coffee creamer
1 tablespoon powdered coffee creamer
1 teaspoon very finely ground, dried culinary lavender
Dash of salt

Blend all ingredients and place in a small zipper-type bag. Makes 4-5 servings (about 1 cup of mix). To prepare: Place 3 to 3-1/2 tablespoons of mix in a mug and add 3/4 cup boiling water. Stir until blended.

To give as a gift, place the plastic bag filled with mix inside a fabric gift bag (see instructions for gift bags on page 51). Attach instructions for preparing beverage.

Gift basket idea: Place a fabric gift bag of mix in a basket that is filled with paper shred. Add an attractive mug.

Lavender Sugar

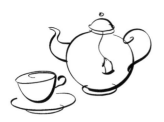

This sugar makes a nice gift when presented in an attractive glass canister with an air-tight, hinged lid.

Place one teaspoon of finely ground, dried culinary lavender and one cup of sugar in a food processor. Process the ingredients to make a fine sugar mixture. Store in an air tight container and use for baking or sweetening tea.

Lavender & Blueberry Pancake Mix

2 cups biscuit mix
1/2 cup dried blueberries,
   chopped
2 tablespoons granulated sugar
2 teaspoons ground, dried
   culinary lavender buds

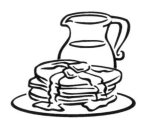

Combine the ingredients until well blended and place in an airtight container or plastic zipper-type bag.

To prepare: Place mix in a large mixing bowl. In a small bowl beat one large egg with 1-1/3 cups of milk. Add egg mixture to pancake mix and stir until smooth and well blended.

Pour about 1/4 cup of batter onto lightly greased hot skillet or griddle. Cook until bubbles appear on top and edges are slightly dry. Turn and cook on the other side until golden brown. Makes about 10 – 12 pancakes.

To give as a gift: Place mix in a plastic zipper-type bag and tuck inside a fabric gift bag. (See page 51 for instructions to make gift bags.) Tie top closed with jute or raffia and attach cooking instructions.

Gift basket idea: Place a fabric gift bag of mix in a basket or skillet that is filled with paper shred. Add a jar of blueberry flavored syrup and a spatula.

Lavender & Peach Scone Mix

2 cups biscuit mix
1/4 cup granulated sugar
2 teaspoons ground, dried
    culinary lavender buds
1 teaspoon dried grated lemon
    peel
3/4 cup dried peaches, very finely chopped

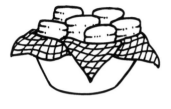

Combine the ingredients until well blended and place in an airtight container or plastic zipper-type bag.

To prepare: Preheat oven to 425°. Place mix in a large mixing bowl. In a small bowl beat one large egg with 1/3 cup of half & half or heavy cream. Add egg mixture to scone mix and stir until well blended.

Turn out onto a lightly floured surface and knead 8-10 times until smooth. Pat or roll dough to 3/4" thickness and cut out circles using a 2-1/2" biscuit cutter. Optional: Brush tops of scones with milk and sprinkle with sugar. Place 1" apart on lightly greased cookie sheet. Bake for 12 to 15 minutes or until golden brown. Makes about 8.

To give as a gift: Place mix in a plastic zipper-type bag and tuck inside a fabric gift bag. (See page 51 for instructions to make gift bags.) Tie top closed with jute or raffia and attach cooking instructions and a biscuit cutter.

Gift basket idea: Place a fabric gift bag of mix in a basket or mixing bowl that is filled with colorful paper shred. Add a biscuit cutter and oven mitt and/or wooden spoon.

If you like, include a bag of Lavender & Cinnamon Spread Mix (page 48) for making flavored butter to serve on the scones.

Creamy Lavender & Potato Soup Mix

1-1/4 cups instant mashed potato flakes
3/4 cup instant nonfat dry milk
1 tablespoon instant chicken bouillon granules
1 teaspoon dried minced onion
1 teaspoon ground dried culinary lavender buds
1 teaspoon dried parsley flakes
1/2 teaspoon seasoned salt
1/4 teaspoon black pepper

Combine all ingredients in a large mixing bowl. Store in an airtight container. Makes about 2 cups of mix.

To prepare: Place 1/2 cup soup mix in a bowl or mug. Add one cup of boiling water. Stir until smooth. Makes one serving.

To give as a gift, place mix in a plastic zipper-type bag and tuck inside a fabric gift bag (see instructions for making gift bags on page 51). Tie bag closed with jute or raffia and attach cooking instructions.

Or place individual servings of soup mix (1/2 cup) into small plastic zipper-type bags. Place one bag in the center of a 12" square of fabric. Gather the fabric around the mix and tie with jute or raffia. Attach cooking instructions. Place inside an attractive mug.

Lavender & Sun Dried Tomato Dip Mix

3 tablespoons sun dried tomatoes, very finely chopped
1 tablespoon ground, dried culinary
    lavender buds
1 tablespoon dried basil leaves, crushed
1 tablespoon dried parsley
1 teaspoon garlic powder
1 teaspoon dried, grated lemon peel
1 teaspoon seasoned salt

Blend all ingredients together and store in an airtight container or small plastic zipper-type bag. Recipe makes about 1/2 cup of mix.

To use: Combine 1 tablespoon of dip mix with 1 cup of sour cream. Add salt and pepper to taste. Chill at least one hour to blend flavors. Serve with chips or fresh vegetables. This dip also tastes great when served on baked potatoes.

To give as a gift, place mix in a small plastic zipper-type bag. Place bag of mix in the center of a 12" square of fabric. Gather the fabric around the mix and tie with jute or raffia. Attach instructions for preparing and serving. Place inside an attractive dip bowl.

Gift basket idea: Place the fabric bundle of dip mix in a basket that is filled with colorful paper shred. Add a bag of chips and a dip bowl.

Lavender & Citrus Marinade Mix

3 tablespoons brown sugar, packed
2 teaspoons ground, dried culinary
    lavender buds
1 teaspoon dried, grated orange peel
1 teaspoon ground cinnamon
1/2 teaspoon salt
1/4 teaspoon ground black pepper

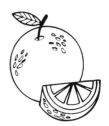

Blend all ingredients together and store in an airtight container or small plastic zipper-type bag. Recipe makes about 1/4 cup of mix.

To use: Combine 1 tablespoon of marinade mix with 1/4 cup of vegetable or olive oil and 1/4 cup of orange juice. Use to marinate beef, chicken or pork for at least one hour before grilling or roasting.

To give as a gift, place mix in a small plastic zipper-type bag. Place bag of mix in the center of a 12" square of fabric. Gather the fabric around the mix and tie with jute or raffia. Attach instructions for preparing and using marinade.

Gift basket idea: Place the fabric bundle of marinade mix in a basket that is filled with colorful paper shred. Add a meat thermometer, pair of tongs and an oven mitt.

Lavender & Almond Rice Seasoning Mix

1/2 cup slivered almonds
3 tablespoons instant chicken bouillon granules
3 tablespoons dried parsley flakes
1 tablespoon instant minced onion
1 tablespoon ground, dried culinary lavender buds
2 teaspoons dried, grated lemon peel
1 teaspoon seasoned salt
1/2 teaspoon ground black pepper

Blend all ingredients together and store in an airtight container or small plastic zipper-type bag. Recipe makes about 1 cup of mix.

To prepare: In a medium saucepan, combine 1 cup of uncooked rice, 2 cups water, 3 tablespoons seasoning mix and 1 tablespoon butter or margarine. Bing to a boil, cover and reduce heat to simmer. Cook 20-25 minutes or until all liquid is absorbed and rice is tender.

To give as a gift, place mix in a small plastic zipper-type bag and tuck inside a fabric gift bag (see instructions on page 51 for making gift bags). Tie top closed with jute or raffia and attach cooking instructions.

Lavender Beer Bread Mix

3 cups self-rising flour
1/3 cup granulated sugar
2 teaspoons ground, dried culinary lavender buds

Combine ingredients and place in a plastic zipper-type bag.

To prepare: Preheat oven to 350°. Grease and flour a 9" X 5" loaf pan. Place mix in large bowl and add one 12 oz. can of beer (at room temperature) and 2 tablespoons of melted butter or margarine. Blend just until ingredients are moistened. Pour into prepared loaf pan. Bake for about 50 minutes or until done. Remove from pan and cool on a wire rack.

To give as a gift, place bag of mix in a fabric gift bag (see instructions on page 51 for making gift bags). Tie top closed with jute or raffia and attach cooking instructions.

Gift basket idea: Place fabric bag of mix inside a small basket or loaf pan that is filled with paper shred. Add a can of beer and a pot holder or oven mitt.

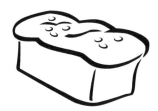

Lavender Spiced Honey

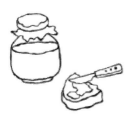

4 cups honey
1 teaspoon ground, dried culinary
    lavender buds
1/2 teaspoon ground cloves
4 cinnamon sticks

Combine honey, lavender and cloves in a saucepan. Add cinnamon sticks and heat over medium heat until very warm (do not boil). Transfer one cinnamon stick to each of four 1/2-pint jars. Fill jars with honey, cover and let stand 24 hours to blend flavors. Store at room temperature for up to three weeks. Use on biscuits, cornbread or pancakes, and to sweeten tea or in any recipes that call for honey.

To give as a gift, cover lid with an 8" square of fabric and secure with a length of raffia around the base of the lid. Tie on a wooden honey dipper.

Lavender & Cinnamon Spread Mix

1/2 cup brown sugar, firmly packed
1 tablespoon ground, dried culinary lavender buds
2 teaspoons ground cinnamon

Blend ingredients together and store in an airtight container or small plastic zipper-type bag. To use: Combine 2 tablespoons of mix with 1 cup of softened cream cheese OR 1/2 cup softened unsalted butter. Chill at least one hour to blend flavors. Soften for 15-20 minutes before serving. Use on bagels, muffins, scones or biscuits.

To give as a gift, place bag of mix in a fabric gift bag (see instructions on page 51 for making gift bags). Tie top closed with jute or raffia and attach instructions.

Lavender & Apple Walnut Muffin Mix

2 cups self-rising flour
1/2 cup granulated sugar
1/4 cup brown sugar, firmly packed
1/2 cup chopped walnuts
2 teaspoons ground, dried culinary
    lavender buds
1 teaspoon ground cinnamon
1 cup dried apples, finely chopped

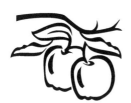

Combine ingredients and place in a plastic, zipper-type bag. Makes about 4 cups of mix.

To prepare: Preheat oven to 400°. Lightly grease 12 muffin cups. In a large bowl, combine muffin mix, one slightly beaten egg, 3/4 cup milk and 1/4 cup vegetable oil. Stir just until moistened. Fill muffin cups 3/4 full. Bake about 15 to 18 minutes or until done.

To give as a gift, place bag of mix inside a fabric gift bag (see instructions for making gift bags on page 51). Tie top closed with raffia and attach a small wooden spoon and cooking instructions.

Gift basket idea: Place fabric bag of mix inside a basket or mixing bowl that is filled with colorful paper shred. Add two pot holders and a wooden spoon.

If you like, include a bag of Lavender & Cinnamon Spread Mix (page 48) for making flavored butter to serve on the apple muffins.

Lavender Chocolate Fudge

Stir up a batch of decadent lavender chocolate fudge and place in a pretty tin or box to give as a gift to a friend or co-worker. They will marvel over the exotic floral flavor.

2 cups (one 12-oz. pkg.) semi-sweet chocolate chips
1 (14 oz.) can sweetened condensed milk
2 teaspoons ground, dried culinary lavender buds
Dash of salt
1/2 cup chopped pecans
1 teaspoon vanilla extract

Grind lavender in a clean coffee grinder before measuring.

In a small, microwave-safe bowl, heat chocolate chips, condensed milk and salt together in the microwave on high power for 1 minute. Stir and then heat an additional 30 seconds if needed. Do not allow to boil. Stir until smooth and all chips are melted.

Stir in lavender, pecans and vanilla. Pour into an 8" square pan lined with foil. Chill until firm then cut into 1" squares.

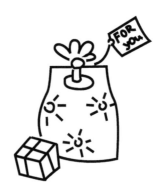

Fabric Gift Bags

To make fabric gift bags, cut two pieces of fabric:

5" wide X 7" high	(for 1/2 cup of mix)
5-1/2" wide X 8-1/2" high	(for 1 cup of mix)
6" wide X 10" high	(for 2 cups of mix)
6-1/2" wide X 11-1/2" high	(for 3 cups of mix)
7" wide X 13" high	(for 4 cups of mix)

Pin the two pieces of fabric together, right sides facing each other. Sew (either by hand or machine) around the sides and bottom of the bag using a 1/4" seam allowance.

To hem the top edge of the bag: Turn the top edge of the bag down 1/4" and press with an iron. Turn the pressed edge down again 1/4" and press. Stitch the hem in place close to the bottom folded edge.

Turn the bag right side out. Add the plastic bag of mix. Gather the top of the fabric bag together just above the bag of mix and tie with raffia, jute or ribbon to close.

Note: If you cut the fabric pieces using pinking shears, pin the two pieces of fabric together, wrong sides facing each other, then sew around the sides and bottom using a 1/4" seam allowance, and you won't need to turn the bag right side out or hem the top.

The Joy of Lavender

Lavender is a beautiful and fragrant herb that has many uses for home and bath.

Potpourris and sachets add a wonderful fragrance to your environment. Sleep pillows and soothing baths help promote relaxation.

And don't forget about the culinary possibilities for making delectable treats and mixes with an exotic floral flavor.

Experiment with the craft projects and recipes in this book to spark your creativity and tickle your senses with lavender.

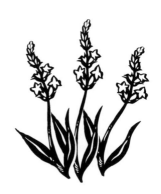

Index

Ordering Information for Dried Herbs

If you don't plan to grow your own lavender and don't have a local source for buying it, you can find many mail-order sources through the Internet. Simply type the words "dried lavender" into your search engine to get a list of companies that sell lavender and other herbs and spices.

I have used the following sources:

San Francisco Herb Company
1-800-227-4530
www.sfherb.com

- dried lavender for cooking & crafting
- dried culinary rose petals
- many other dried herbs for crafting
- a wide variety of dried spices
- muslin drawstring bags for bath herbs
- small plastic zipper-type bags
- flax seed for eye pillows

Mountain Rose Herbs
1-800-879-3337
www.mountainroseherbs.com

- dried lavender for cooking & crafting
- lavender flower powder
- dried rose petals and rose powder
- herbal tea blends & tea brewing bags
- many other dried herbs for crafting
- a wide variety of dried spices
- muslin drawstring bags for bath herbs
- wooden scoops
- flax seed for eye pillows

About the Author

Gloria Hander Lyons has channeled 30 years of training and hands-on experience in the areas of art, interior decorating, crafting and event planning into writing creative how-to books. Her books cover a wide range of topics including decorating your home, cooking, planning weddings and tea parties, crafting and self-publishing.

She has designed original needlework and craft projects featured in magazines, such as *Better Homes and Gardens, McCall's, Country Handcrafts* and *Crafts*.

She teaches interior decorating, self-publishing and wedding planning classes at her local community college. Much to her family's delight, her kitchen is in non-stop test mode, creating recipes for new cookbooks.

Visit her website: www.BlueSagePress.com

Other Books by Gloria Hander Lyons

- *Easy Microwave Desserts in a Mug*
- *Easy Microwave Desserts in a Mug for Kids*
- *No Rules – Just Fun Decorating*
- *Just Fun Decorating for Tweens & Teens*
- *If Teapots Could Talk: Fun Ideas for Tea Parties*
- *The Super-Bride's Guide for Dodging Wedding Pitfalls*
- *Designs That Sell: How To Make Your Home Show Better and Sell Faster*
- *A Taste of Lavender: Delectable Treats with an Exotic Floral Flavor*
- *Self-Publishing on a Budget: A Do-It-All-Yourself Guide*
- *The Secret Ingredient: Tasty Recipes with an Unusual Twist*
- *Hand Over the Chocolate & No One Gets Hurt! The Chocolate-Lover's Cookbook*

Ordering Information

To order additional copies of this book, send check or money order payable to:

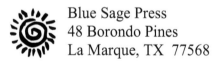 Blue Sage Press
48 Borondo Pines
La Marque, TX 77568

Cost for this edition is $6.95 per book (U.S. currency only) plus $3.00 shipping and handling for the first book and $1.25 for each additional book shipped to the same U.S. address.

Texas residents add 8.25% sales tax to total order amount.

To pay by credit card or get a complete list of books written by Gloria Hander Lyons, visit our website at:

www.BlueSagePress.com.

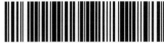
7653161R00035

Printed in Great Britain
by Amazon.co.uk, Ltd.,
Marston Gate.